How to lose weight

a simple and effective approach to weight loss & fat loss

———————————

How to lose weight.
Copyright © 2019 by Mark Chatham

ISBN (978-0-244-81432-8)

Table of Contents

Foreword

Before starting a diet or work-out program, please consult your doctor to ensure you are capable of following both the diet and the work-out programs. If at any point during the diet or work-out programs you become ill or get injured, please stop the program and consult your doctor immediately.

Chapter One: The Book

Why Write This Book?

People need help losing weight and reaching their targets. This book aims to provide that help.

Approach Of This Book

The concept for this book is to provide a small, easy to understand, and easy to follow book that will tell you how to lose fat and get you started on your journey of fat loss.

The book takes a "straight-to-the-point" approach, with small chapters giving just the key information you actually need. At the end of the book is a **Further Information** section, which provides you with further details on various topics.

This approach will allow you to get the information you need to get started, straight away. Then as time passes you can gain a more detailed understanding of a topic and use this increased knowledge to fine tune your approach.

Why Do You Need A Book?

You don't!

To lose fat, you do not need this or any book. Everyday people successfully lose fat, but too often they hit problems which delay or completely stop them from reaching their targets.

This book intends to give you the information to allow you to create an approach which will get you results, longer-term health benefits, and provide you with success on your fat loss journey.

We often require someone else to tell us what we already know! It give us confidence to do what we know we should do, and how we should do it. This book aims to give you the confidence to start your journey to a learner, healthier, and happier you!

Why Should You Trust This Book?

Because the book is based on the knowledge gained from being where you are now and reaching where you will get to.

Going from 260lbs to 125lbs, and eventually getting to a stable 150lbs. During this process, at points starving and losing muscle, and falling off the process too many times!

This book can help you avoid those mistakes, and help to get you to your target quicker.

So How Much Will This Cost?

Just the cost of this book! Nothing else, no programs, no subscriptions, no useless equipment, no branded supplements, no branded clothing!

You just need to give 100% effort, be 100% honest with yourself, and give 100% commitment. In return this may change your life and make you the person you desire.

100% effort!
100% honesty!
100% commitment!

Book Structure

This book is split into the following sections: Chapter 2, gives an overview of how fat loss works; Chapter 3, documents how to approach your fat loss; Chapter 4, sets your starting point; Chapter 5, gives you an overview of your diet approach; Chapter 6, gives an overview of the cardio approach; Chapter 7, gives an overview of the weight-lifting approach; Chapter 8, sets the approach for NEAT; Chapter 9, discusses sleep requirements; Chapter 10, discusses fitting the approach into your life; Chapter 11, discusses measuring your progress; Chapter 12, provides some tips; then, there is the further information section, and finally details of support.

Now What?

Now...you take a deep breath. Then you turn the page. Then you start reading. But most importantly you start your journey...now!

Start now...not tomorrow, not on Monday,

not next week, not next month, not January 1st – But NOW!

The sooner you start your journey, the sooner you will start to see progress, the sooner the momentum will grow, the sooner you reach your target.

Chapter 2: How Fat Lose Works

Why Lose Fat?

We want to lose fat. Not water weight. Not muscle. But just fat. Why? Losing fat will increase your heath and aid the re-composition of your body (from where it is now, to a leaner and more muscular physique).

How Body Weight Works

Let's go through the basics of how body weight works. This will be all the information you need to start losing fat (further information is available at the back of the book or any one of a thousand other books or any one of a thousand websites...but you do **not** need more information).

Your body (body weight) works on Calories (Cals or Kcals). Calories, are a unit of measurement for energy to fuel your activities. All the food **and** all the drinks (*yes, drinks as well*) you consume have calories (there are a few exceptions e.g. water which has 0 calories):

These calories control if you put on weight!

These calories control if you lose weight!

These calories control if you stay the same weight!

Furthermore, these calories also decide the composition of the body (muscle vs. fat):

These calories control if you build muscle!

These calories control if you lose muscle!

These calories control if you add fat to your body!

These calories control if you lose fat from your body!

What Does The Body Use Calories For?

Your body uses the calories you consume (*and the calories stored in the fat within your body*) as an **energy source** to keep you alive and fuel your activities. The activities your body performs include:

Task	Meaning	Comment
BMR	Basal Metabolic Rate	All the bodily functioning used at rest, e.g. breathing, beating heart, growing skin, growing hair, pumping blood, brain activity, etc.
TEF	Thermic Effect of Food	Chewing food, breaking-down food, increase in body temperature, increase in metabolic rate.
NEAT	Non-Exercise Activity Thermogenesis	Activities which are non-exercised, e.g. gardening, work, dusting, etc.
EAT	Exercise Activity Thermogenesis	Exercising activities e.g. running, swimming, weight-lifting, etc.

The breakdown of how much each of these activities take of your daily calorie intake is surprising, with between 55% and 85% consumed by just the BMR.

Task	Comment	Estimated Percentage	
		Low activity person	High activity person
BMR	All tasks to keep your body functioning at rest.	85%	55%
TEF	Thermic effect of food (energy to consume food)	10%	10%
NEAT	Non-Exercise activity thermogenesis e.g. day-to-day activities like gardening.	5%	20%
EAT	Exercise activity thermogenesis e.g. going for a run or walking	0%	15%

Calories In

All of the calories you consume are added together each day, to make your **Calories In** (*the number of calories you have consumed that day*).

Various governments have recommendations for daily calorie intake know as Recommend Daily Activities (RDA) or Guideline Daily Activities (GDA), generally these are:

Person	RDA / GDA
Child (Female & Male)	1500
Adult (Female)	2000
Adult (Male)	2500

Remember these are just guidelines, and are not accurate. The calorie requirement for a 23 year old woman who weights 120 lbs and is very active is **not** going to be the same as the calorie requirements of a 55 year old woman who weighs 120 lbs but is not active and is **not** going to be the same as the calorie requirements of a 30 year old woman who is 200 lbs.

Calories Out

The activities your body performs each day are your **Calories Out** (*the number of calories your body needs to perform activities*). This is known as your Total Daily Energy Expenditure (TDEE).

Each day your **Calories Out** will be different due to the amount of sleep, activity, exercise, etc. you have performed that day.

Two people doing the exact same activities in a day but weighing different amounts or of different ages, will have different calories out (TDEE) that day.

Fat Loss Basics

Now we have simplified **Calories In** and **Calories Out**. We can start to discuss how this affects fat loss.

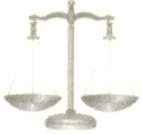

Fat loss (or fat gain or staying at the same fat level) is determined by the number of calories in **versus** the number of calories out.

Think of it as a Balance Scale. On one side is your calories in and on the other side your calories out.

Scenario 1: If your [Calories In] is **more** than your [Calories Out] – you will gain fat. In this scenario you are eating more calories than you need to perform your activities. *This is fat gain*. **This is bad and not what you want to happen**.

Scenario 2: If your [Calories In] is **less** than your [Calories Out] – you will lose fat. In this scenario you are eating less calories than you need to perform your activities. *This is called fat loss*. **This is what you want to happen**.

Scenario 3: If your [Calories In] is **the same** as your [Calories Out] – you will not lose and not gain fat. In this scenario you are eating the same amount of calories as you need to perform your activities.

This is a simplistic view of fat loss and fat gain, and is at a very high-level. But the concept is accurate for your approach.

This book is all about a simple approach, therefore the key thing for you to remember is:

[Calories In] less than [Calories Out] equals fat loss.

How Do You Create Fat Loss

As discussed, to get fat loss you just need your [Calories In] (the calories you have consumed) to be **less** than your [Calories Out] (the calories you have used). We need to create a **deficit** where [Calories In] is less than [Calories Out]. Mathematically:

$$Fat\ Loss = ([Calories\ In] < [Calories\ Out])$$

What Are Calories?

Calories are made-up of **Macronutrients**. There are four basic types of macronutrients:-

- Carbohydrates.
- Protein.
- Fat.
- Alcohol.

What Are Macronutrients

Macronutrients are larger nutrients (there are also smaller nutrients called Micronutrients) which are substances that are needed by your body to perform house-keeping (growing, performing bodily functions, etc.)

When you consume the macronutrients the body transforms them, so as to be able to effectively provide energy for your body to use.

What are Micronutrients

Micronutrients are often referred to as vitamins and minerals which are required by your body. Micronutrients cannot be produced by your body so must be included in your diet.

Not All Macronutrients Are Equal

Not all the macronutrients have the same energy value per 1 gram. The calories per one gram of the each macronutrient is as follows:

Macronutrient	Calories per 1 gram
Fat	9
Ethanol (alcohol)	7
Carbohydrates	4
Protein	4

As you can see Fat is the most calorie dense macronutrient at 9 calories per 1 gram of fat. Then Alcohol is the next calorie dense macronutrient at 7 calories per 1 gram of alcohol. Then Carbohydrates and Protein each at 4 calories per 1 gram.

How Are Calories Calculated?

A food calorie (Kcal) is calculated as follows:

$$Calories = (fat\ grams * 9) +$$
$$(alcohol\ grams * 7) +$$
$$(carbohydrate\ grams * 4) +$$
$$(protein\ grams * 4)$$

So if we have a food source that has 10 grams of Fat, 1 gram of Alcohol, 16 grams of Carbohydrates, and 3 grams of Protein. We get:

$$Calories = (10g * 9) + (1g * 7) +$$
$$(16g * 4) + (3g * 4)$$
$$Calories = (90) + (7) + (64) + (12)$$
$$Calories = 173$$

Body's Fuel Sources

The body has three main sources of fuel that it can use:

Priority	Fuel Source	Comment
1	Food and drinks consumed	Good source to use.
2	Body's stored fat	Good source to use.
3	Body's stored muscle	Bad source to use.

The primary source of fuel (to provide the energy you use to perform your activities) is the food and drinks you consume.

If the food and drinks you consume is not enough to fuel your activities, the body will then use stored fat for energy – which is what you want to happen so you lose fat.

If you consume so little food and drinks for a long period (starvation) your body will have consumed enough stored fat to be at a low body fat %, and will then start to use your muscles as fuel – **a very bad thing for your body**. *We need to ensure this does not happen.*

Why Use Stored Fat?

Using your stored fat to fuel your energy will reduce your stored fat levels, which will reduce your body fat percentage (%), and aid your body re-composition.

Calories In 1 Pound (lb) Of Fat

As a rough rule-of-thumb there are 3500 [Calories In] 1 pound (lb) of Fat (0.45 kilograms). So if you want to lose 1 lb of fat across 1 week you could reduce [Calories In] by 500 or increase your [Calories Out] by 500 or reduce your [Calories In] by 250 & increase your [Calories Out] by 250.

That 500 difference over 7 days would add upto 3500 calories or 1 lb of fat.

Chapter 3: Your Approach

Your Approach To Fat Loss

This chapter gives an overview of how you will approach your fat loss.

Create An Deficit

As you read in Chapter 2, fat loss occurs when the amount of calories you have consumed (your [Calories In]) is **less** than the number of calories you have used in activities (your [Calories Out]).

The bigger the deficit between your [Calories In] and your [Calories Out], then the larger the fat loss.

So what will you do to ensure there is a deficit between your [Calories In] and [Calories Out]? There are three approaches you can take:

- Scenario 1: Reduce the calories you consume, by eating a little less (**reduce [Calories In]**).

- Scenario 2: Increase the calories you use, by doing a little more activity (**increase [Calories Out]**).

Scenario 3: Reduce the calories you consume (**reduce [Calories In]**)

&

increase the calories you use (**increase [Calories Out]**), by eating a little less and by doing a little more activity.

How To Reduce [Calories In]

You will reduce the calories you consume, simply by eating less calories (although not necessary less food). This can be done by reducing the calories you eat from 2500 calories a day to eating 2250 calories a day. This 250 calorie a day reduction over a 7 day period will total to 1750 calories, meaning you will lose around 0.5 lb of fat per week.

By substituting foods, e.g. rather than eating a chocolate bar (200 – 250 kcals) instead eating a banana (100 – 150 kcals) you have achieved three things:

1. Reduced calories in by 100 calories.

2. Eaten 50g more volume of food (100g-150g banana) instead of 50g chocolate bar.

3. Provided micronutrients to your body.

The end result of doing this will also keep you fuller for longer and get your body performing better.

How To Increase [Calories Out]

You will increase the calories you used, simply by doing more. You can do this by the following methods:-

- Increase your **NEAT** activities: Do this by either doing some or doing more, general activities, e.g. gardening or washing your car or hoovering or dusting. Just increase your activity tasks.
- Increase your **EAT** activities: Do this by starting an exercise program or increasing your current exercise program.
- Increase your **BMR**: Do this by increasing your muscle mass. This is a slow process and will take months to build muscle (0.5 to 1 pound of muscle per month), but this increase in muscle mass will increase your BMR by around 8 calories per day per additional pound of muscle mass.
- Increase **Themogenesis effect**: Your body needs to be kept at a temperature between 97°F (36.1°C) and 99°F (37.2°C), (averaging 98.6°F (37°C)). If your are too cold your body will burn calories to increase your temperature; if your body is too hot your body will burn calories to reduce your temperature. **This approach is not discussed further.**

So how are you going to increase your [Calories Out]. Simple! You will be doing more NEAT activity, you will be doing more EAT and indirectly by food choices and EAT you will increase your BMR and thermogensis effect from working out.

Your Approach

The approach you will take is to reduce your [Calories In] **and** increase your [Calories Out].

The next few chapters (from Chapter 5 – 8) will focus on cardio (increasing your [Calories Out]), weight-lifting (increasing your [Calories Out] and increasing your muscle mass), NEAT activities (increasing your [Calories Out]), and also via diet (reducing your [Calories In]).

An approach of both reducing [Calories In] **and** increasing [Calories Out], offers the fastest way to get to your goal. On top of this, it also offers longer-term benefits:-

- Over time, the cardio activities (EAT) will increase your aerobic capacity, which will offer you better overall fitness. This will also make your body more efficient at consuming calories.

- The NEAT activities will give you less time to focus on food, and improve your mental health, by keeping you focused.

- Weight-lifting (EAT) will increase your muscle mass which will improve your body re-composition (going from a larger body image to a leaner body image). The additional muscle mass you build will also help reduce your body fat percentage, as the muscle percentage is increasing whilst the fat percentage is decreasing.

- Diet will help your performance at EAT.

Target (Approach)

You should aim for 1 to 3 lbs (0.45 to 1.36 kgs) of body fat loss per week. This will be between a 500 and 1500 calorie difference per day. We will divide this number into diet, cardio, weight-lifting, and NEAT.

- Target for diet is 50% of the calorie difference.

- Target for cardio is 30% of the calorie difference.

- Target for weight-lifting is 10% of the calorie difference.

- Target for NEAT is 10% of the calorie difference.

Target Fat Loss Per week	Diet changes per day (50%)	Cardio per day (30%)	Weight-lifiting per day (10%)	NEAT per day (10%)
0.5 lbs (0.22 kg)	Reduce by 125 calories	Do 75 calories	Do 25 calories	Do 25 calories
1lbs (0.45 kg)	Reduce by 250 calories	Do 150 calories	Do 50 calories	Do 50 calories
1.5 lbs (0.68 kg)	Reduce by 375 calories	Do 225 calories	Do 75 calories	Do 75 calories
2 lbs (0.90 kg)	Reduce by 500 calories	Do 300 calories	Do 100 calories	Do 100 calories
2.5 lbs (1.13 kg)	Reduce by 625 calories	Do 375 calories	Do 125 calories	Do 125 calories
3 lbs (1.36 kg)	Reduce by 750 calories	Do 450 calories	Do 150 calories	Do 150 calories

Calorie Difference Warning

WARNING: Always ensure you consume a minimum of between 1200 and 1800 calories per day. If you consume less than 1200 to 1800 calories over a period of time this will cause your BMR to drop by a large amount and cause you permanent health problems.

Chapter 4: Your Starting Point

Starting Point

Everyone who uses this book to achieve their goals will be starting from a different position, have different amounts of fat to lose, and have different goals and milestones, therefore you need to set your own starting point.

Setting Your Starting Point

You need to take measurements at your starting point. The measurements you should record are:

1. Recording your weight in pounds (lbs).

2. Recording your waist circumference (around the belly-button) in centimeters (cm).

3. Recording your Hip circumference (widest point) in centimeters (cm).

4. Photos, showing front, side, and back pictures of your body. *Depending on where your starting point is and how comfortable you are doing this.*

   Whatever your starting point is, write it down! Now!

Setting Your Target

Once you have your starting point, you next need to set you target. This may be as simple as setting an amount of weight you want to lose or size to get to.

Whatever your target is, write it down! Now!

Setting Your Timescales

Once you know your starting point and you know your target, it is just a case of working out your timescale. The easiest approach for this is to subtract your target from your starting point.

Your starting weight is 250 lbs.

Your target weight is 180 lbs.

You have to lose 70 lbs.

Once you have the amount to lose you can then roughly plan this out. Start with 2 lbs per a week. 2 lbs of fat loss usually reduces waist by 0.25 cm to 0.50 cm.

70 lbs divided by 2 lbs (per week) is 35 weeks.

Once you have the number of weeks add 25% - 50% contingency. Extra contingency is important as you will hit problems.

*35 weeks * 1.25 (25% extra) = 44 weeks.*

*35 weeks * 1.50 (50% extra) = 53 weeks.*

Although your final figure may be larger than you want it to be, it is better to be realistic with your plan than to start an unrealistic plan and fail!

Chapter 5: Your Diet

Diet

What is a diet? A way to lose fat? – **NO!**

Diet means "regular way of life" (in classical Greek) and you **must** think of your diet as something you will continue after you reach your target.

Your Diet Approach

You will approach this diet as a **way of life** where you will make three small changes which together will make big differences:

1. Replace poorer nutritional foods for better nutritional foods. For example, replacing fried chips for steamed potatoes. *This will get your body functioning better for longer-term health benefits and reduce the calories you consume.*

2. Replace low-volume & high-calorie foods (chocolate, cake, biscuits, etc.) with high-volume & low-calorie foods (fruit, vegetables, etc.) For example, replacing chocolate (around 500 calories per 100g) for bananas (around 100 calories per 100g). *This will keep you filled up, and reduce your calories consumed.*

3. Reduce your calories consumed. For example, replacing 4 sausages with 3 sausages; removing mayonnaise from tuna sandwich. *This will reduce the calories you are eating.*

Overview Of Types Of Diets

There are an endless number of diets for you to choose from. These can range from ultra-clean food diets, to dirty food diets, to simple food reduction, to food substitutions, to limited foods only...the possibilities are endless. The short-term results will be similar, however over the longer term, different diets offer better longer-term health benefits.

Name	Description	Weight loss?	Positives	Negatives	Ease to follow	Longer term health benefits	Risks
Limited Food Diet.	These diets are where you are limited by either the food (e.g. cauliflower only diet) or the types of foods (e.g. Protein – Steak and Egg diet) or the prepared food (e.g. Cauliflower Soup diet).	Yes *	Routine based	Limited food choices. Need strong will power.	Starts easy gets harder	Not many.	Health risks from limited diet.
Clean Food Diet.	These diets are where you eat only "clean" foods (generally speaking non-processed natural foods like fruit, vegetables, meat, and grains).	Yes *	Choice of food. Micronutrients available from food.	Cost of foods can be higher.	Starts tough, can become a routine.	Increased health benefits	N/a.
Dirty Food Diet.	These diets allow you to eat whatever you want (e.g. Cakes, Biscuits, Crisps, Chips, etc.) but reduced amount.	Yes *	Same foods as currently eat.	Foods used to. Cheaper to purchase.	Starts easy, but need control to avoid over-eating.	Not many.	Over-eating and putting on weight.
Fasting Diet.	Going with little or no food for periods. Either x hours each days or x number of days a week.	Yes *	Same foods as currently eat.	Periods of hunger.	Starts tough, can become a routine.	Some.	Not so alert.

Quiz Time

What have you learned? Hopefully you have learned: whatever diet you choose, if you eat less calories than you burn (your [Calories In] is **less** than your [Calories Out]) then you will lose fat.

All you need to remember to lose fat:

Eat less calories than you use!

How Do Diets Work

All diets work the same way, reducing the number of calories consumed results in fat loss. For example, lets take the 5:2 diet where a person eats 2500 calories for 5 days and 500 calories for 2 days. If we assume that the person needs 2500 calories per day, on the two days they eat 500 calories, they have a 2000 calorie reduction per day (4000 calorie over the week). This 4000 calorie reduction is the fat loss.

Now assume the same person reduced there daily calories by 571 calories (4000 / 7), so they consume 1929 calories each day. Over the week they will have reduced their calories by 4000 calories which will be the **same** fat loss.

What Diet Should You Choose?

We will call your diet, the **replace & reduce** diet. It will consist of doing two things:

- Replace some foods with healthier foods.

- Reduce the amount of calories you consume.

Now, lets start looking at real examples, of replacing and reducing.

Replace & Reduce Examples

Below are examples of an average persons meals, and the substitutions and reductions that can be applied:

Meal	Current	Replacement	Reduction	Estimated Calorie reduction
Breakfast	Granola & semi-skimmed Milk	50g of porridge & water		150 – 200
Breakfast	4 Slices of Toast & Butter	No butter		50 – 75
Breakfast	50g of porridge & water		40g of porridge & water	40
Breakfast	4 Slices of Toast & Jam		3 Slices of Toast & Jam	75 – 110
Breakfast	Scrambled Eggs (made with Milk) & 4 Toasts	Microwave Eggs (with Water) & 4 Toasts		50
Breakfast	Microwave Eggs (with Water) & 4 Toasts		Microwave Eggs (with Water) & 3 Toasts	50 -100
Breakfast	4 x Sausage, Bacon, Fried Bread, Baked Beans,	4 x Sausage, Toast, Tomatoes		100 – 200
Breakfast	4 x Sausage, Toast, Tomatoes		2 x Sausage, Toast, Tomatoes	200 -300

Meal	Current	Replacement	Reduction	Estimated Calorie reduction
Lunch	Cheese Sandwich (Cheese; White Bread; Butter; Pickle)	Ham Salad (Brown Bread; Lettuce)		200 – 250
Lunch	Ham Sandwich (White Bread; Butter; Tomato Sauce)	Ham (Brown Bread; Lettuce; Tomato)		100 – 200
Lunch	Tuna Salad (Tuna in Oil; Mayonnaise)	Use Tuna in Spring Water or Tuna in Brine instead		100
Lunch	Tuna Salad (Tuna in Oil; Mayonnaise)		Remove Mayonnaise	100
Lunch	Pizza (3 Slices)		Pizza (2 Slices)	150 – 300
Lunch	Hamburger & Chips	Hamburger		200
Lunch	Hamburger	Chicken Burger (Grilled Chicken not breading)		100

Meal	Current	Replacement	Reduction	Estimated Calorie reduction
Dinner	4 Sausages, Chips & Baked Beans.	Boiled Potatoes instead of Chips.		100
Dinner	4 Sausages, Chips & Baked Beans.		3 Sausages instead of 4 Sausages. Reduce the amount of Baked Beans.	150
Dinner	Lasagne (Beef, Tomatoes, Cheese, Cheese Sauce, Pasta Sheets)	Lasagne (Lean Beef, Tomatoes, Mushrooms, Pasta Sheets)		200 – 300
Dinner	Spaghetti Bolognaise	Tuna Pasta with no sauces (Homemade)		200
Dinner	Spaghetti Bolognaise	Tomato, Mushroom, Spinach Pasta (Homemade)		200 – 300
Dinner	Fried Steak, Fried Chips, Sauce	Grilled Steak, Boiled Potatoes		200 – 300

Meal	Current	Replacement	Reduction	Estimated Calorie reduction
Pudding	Chocolate Pudding.		Smaller serving	50 – 100
Pudding	Chocolate Pudding.	Fruit instead of Chocolate Pudding.		100 – 150
Pudding	Strawberry Yoghurt	Natural low fat Yoghurt		50 – 75
Pudding	Cheesecake	2 Rice Cakes & Cottage Cheese		150 – 300
Pudding	Cheesecake		Smaller portion	50 – 100
Pudding	Pancakes, Ice Cream		Pancakes (no Ice Cream)	100 – 150
Pudding	Ice Cream	Ice Sorbet		100 – 150

Meal	Current	Replacement	Reduction	Estimated Calorie reduction
Snack	Chocolate Bar		Half a chocolate bar	100
Snack	Chocolate Bar	Banana		50 – 75
Snack	Bag of crisps		Half a bag of crisps	50
Snack	Bag of crisps	3 Rice Cakes		100
Snack	Chocolate Biscuit	1 Rice Cake		25
Snack	5 Chocolate Biscuits		3 Chocolate Biscuits	100 – 150

Meal	Current	Replacement	Reduction	Estimated Calorie reduction
Drink	Tea, milk, & biscuit	Black tea with no biscuit		50 – 75
Drink	Coffee, milk, & biscuit	Black coffee with no biscuit		50 – 75
Drink	Tea with milk	Black tea		25
Drink	Coffee with milk	Black coffee		25
Drink	Pint of Cola	Pint of calorie-free cola		150
Drink	Pint of Cola	Pint of Water		150
Drink	Orange Juice	Low-calorie orange squash		100 – 150
Drink	Orange Juice	Water		200

Why Replace?

Why replace? Why not just reduce? This is a good question to ask. You could of course just eat less amounts of your current diet and this will result in you losing fat.

But the point of replacing is to improve the foods you eat. The improvement is two-fold:

1. Getting more volume (grams of food) for less calories. For example 100 grams of oven chips is around 175 calories, whilst 190 grams of steamed potatoes is around 175 calories. So for the same calories you get to eat 90 grams more food.

2. Getting better nutrient foods. By replacing a chocolate bar for a banana, you will get micronutrients.

This replacement to increase volume will ensure you are kept 'full', so you are less hungry. The replacement to better nutrient foods will help to ensure you body performs better. Everything from working-out...to reading...to sleeping...to going to the toilet.

Example Meals

Below are some examples meals to get you started:

Meal	Details	Estimated Calories
Breakfast	50g of porridge & water.	200
Breakfast	50g of porridge & water. Banana.	300
Breakfast	4 x Medium Brown Bread (no butter)	200 – 300
Breakfast	4 x Medium Brown Bread With a Banana	300 – 400
Breakfast	50g of Natural Yoghurt, 100g Mixed Frozen Berries	300 – 400
Breakfast	2 Eggs boiled, 2 slices of Brown Bread, 3 tomatoes	400 – 450
Breakfast	4 Eggs scrambled cooked in Microwave with water (no milk or butter)	300

Meal	Details	Estimated Calories
Lunch	Lettuce, Tuna (in Brine), Tomato, Cucumber, Carrots. **No dressing.**	300 – 400
Lunch	Ham Sandwich (4 slices) and Lettuce	300 – 400
Lunch	4 Rice Cakes, 4 Cheese slices, Tomatoes	200 – 300
Lunch	Tuna (in Brine), 300g of mixed Frozen Vegetables	300 – 400
Lunch	Chicken Breast (grilled), Sweet Potato, 100g Broccoli	300 – 400
Lunch	50g Rice, 100g Tomatoes, 200g Mushrooms	300 – 350

Meal	Details	Estimated Calories
Dinner	Fish, 200g Steamed Potatoes, 200g Carrots, 200g Broccoli, 200g Cauliflower	300 – 400
Dinner	Chicken Breast, 200g Potatoes, 300g Broccoli	300 – 400
Dinner	Spaghetti (25g), 100g Tomatoes, 25g Lean Beef, 200g Mushrooms	400 – 500
Dinner	Grilled medium-sized Steak, 200g Potatoes, 200g Mushrooms, 100g Peas	400 – 500
Dinner	Beef Stew (Carrots, Potatoes, Swedes, Turnips, Peas)	300 – 400

Meal	Details	Estimated Calories
Pudding	Fruit Salad 50g	200
Pudding	Yoghurt 50g	100
Pudding	Yoghurt 50g, 100g Mixed Berries	150
Pudding	Sugar Free Low Calorie Jelly (25g)	25 – 100
Pudding	3 Rice Cakes, Banana	200

Meal	Details	Estimated Calories
Snack	Banana (Medium)	100
Snack	Apple	75
Snack	Orange	60
Snack	3 Rice Cakes (plain)	90
Snack	3 Rice Cakes (Chocolate)	120
Snack	3 Rice Cakes (plain) and 10g of Peanut Butter	140

Meal	Details	Estimated Calories
Drink	Pint of Sugar Free Cola	20
Drink	Pint of Blackcurrant Squash	20
Drink	Cup of Coffee **No milk.**	10
Drink	Cup of Tea **No milk.**	10
Drink	Pint of Water	0
Drink	Pint of Sugar Free Cola	20
Drink	Pint of Blackcurrant Squash	20

Next Step

For the next 3 to 5 days, eat normally and write down all the food and drink you consume each day. Then you can use a calorie calculate (see Chapter 12) to work-out the rough average of your total calories for each of those days.

Be 100% honest about this, to ensure you get the most accurate values, and calculate an accurate average.

Daily Meal Split

Initially, we will aim for 6 meals a day. This will be split into 3 main meals (Breakfast, Lunch, and Dinner), and 3 snacks. As time goes by you can revise this to increase or reduce the number of meals you would like (e.g. smaller meals more frequently or larger meals less frequently).

Below is a table of meal splits for 1500 through 3000 calories per a day. This amount is **after** your deduction, e.g. if you currently consume 3000 calories per day and are going to have a 1000 calorie deficit, you would use the 2000 calories column.

Meal	%age of Calories In	Calories In						
		1500	1750	2000	2250	2500	2750	3000
Breakfast	25%	375	438	500	563	625	688	750
Lunch	25%	375	438	500	563	625	688	750
Dinner	20%	300	350	400	450	500	550	600
Snack 1	10%	150	175	200	225	250	275	300
Snack 2	10%	150	175	200	225	250	275	300
Snack 3	10%	150	175	200	225	250	275	300

Meal Timmings

Initially, aim for 3 hour gap between main meals (Breakfast, Lunch, and Dinner) and the following snack. Aim for 2 hours between snacks and the following main meal.

Meal	Timing
Breakfast	
Snack 1	3 hours after Breakfast
Lunch	2 hours after Snack 1
Snack 2	3 hours after Lunch
Dinner	2 hours after Snack 2
Snack 3	2 hours after Dinner

Target (Diet)

You should aim for 1 to 3 lbs (0.45 to 1.36 kgs) of body fat loss per week. This will be between a 500 and 1500 calorie difference per day. For diet the target will be 50% of the calorie difference.

Target Fat Loss per week	Diet changes per day (50%)
0.5 lbs (0.22 kg)	Reduce by **125** calories
1lbs (0.45 kg)	Reduce by **250** calories
1.5 lbs (0.68 kg)	Reduce by **375** calories
2 lbs (0.90 kg)	Reduce by **500** calories
2.5 lbs (1.13 kg)	Reduce by **625** calories
3 lbs (1.36 kg)	Reduce by **750** calories

Calorie Difference Warning

WARNING: Always ensure you consume a minimum of between 1200 and 1800 calories per day. If you consume less than 1200 to 1800 calories over a period of time this will cause your BMR to drop by a large amount and cause you permanent health problems.

Chapter 6: Your Cardio

What Is Cardio

From your point-of-view, consider cardio as an activity you do for the purpose of exercise. Examples of cardio, include:

- Walking at pace.
- Jogging.
- Cycling.
- Sprinting.
- Karate lesson.
- Dance class.
- Playing football.
- Swimming.
- Walking up-and-down stairs for a period of time.

Examples of non-cardio, are listed below. These are NEAT tasks, and are generally day-to-day activities you perform which are not for an exercise purpose:

- Walking to the shops.
- Gardening.
- House work.
- Moving objects around a warehouse.

Your Cardio Approach

Your approach to cardio is based on two simple principles:

1. Consistently performing cardio. *This will be ensuring you consistently keep moving.*

2. Small increments in your cardio. *This will ensure over-time you increase your cardio. Whether it is an increase from 3 days a week, to 4 days a week, to 5 days a week, etc. or from 10 minutes a day, to 15 minutes a day, to 20 minutes a day, etc. or by moving from walking to jogging to sprinting.*

Starting Point

Everybody who reads this book will have their own starting point, whether this is currently doing no cardio at all, or currently doing infrequent cardio, or currently doing cardio twice a week for 20 minutes, or currently doing cardio 5 times a week for 30 minutes.

The first thing for you to do is to write down what cardio you current do, including:

- How often you do the cardio each week.

- How long you do the cardio for per session.

- How intense the cardio is (e.g. leisurely walking to intensely sprinting)

This is now your starting point!

Small Increments

This helps you to focus on regularly making small increments to the cardio you are performing.

This is necessary to do as, when you lose weight and get fitter your body gets more efficient, so you use less calories to perform the same cardio.

As an example someone weighing 200 lbs who cycles for 30 minutes at any average pace may use 125 calories. Now when that person gets to 150 lbs and cycles for the same time at the same pace they use less calories (e.g. 100 calories).

The fitter and healthier you get the more efficient your body becomes. So regular small increments are necessary to maintain the effectiveness of the cardio.

How To Increment

Every period (weekly or monthly) you are simply going to do one (or more) of the following:

1. Increase how frequently you do cardio. Until you are doing cardio 7 days per week.

2. Increase how long you do cardio each day. Up to a maximum of 60 minutes cardio per day.

3. Increase the intensity of the cardio. **Making sure you do not over-do the intensity of your cardio, you do not injury yourself, and you do not impact your mobility.**

Example Increments

Example 1: You currently do no cardio, your first 5 increments could be:

1. Increment to: 5 minutes walking 1 times a week.
2. Increment to: 5 minutes walking 2 days a week.
3. Increment to: 5 minutes walking 3 days a week.
4. Increment to: 5 minutes walking 4 days a week.
5. Increment to: 5 minutes walking 5 days a week.

Example 2: You currently do 7 cardio sessions of 30 minutes cycling a week, your first 3 increments could be:

1. Increment to: 35 minutes cycling 7 days a week.
2. Increment to: 40 minutes cycling 7 days a week.
3. Increment to: 45 minutes cycling 7 days a week.

Example 3: You currently do 7 cardio sessions of 45 minutes running a week, your first 3 increments could be:

1. Increment to: Add 5 minutes skipping rope to 45 minutes running 7 days a week.
2. Increment to: Increase to 10 minutes skipping rope on top of 45 minutes running 7 days a week.
3. Increment to: Increase to 15 minutes skipping rope on top of 45 minutes running 7 days a week.

Why Small Increments?

Small increments are done to ensure you do not over do it, burn-out, or take too much on too quickly and give-up. They also help you to stay motivated.

Keep your increments small and regular.

How Often To Increment

You will be the best person to judge this, but as a guide for larger people currently doing no or little cardio increment slowly at first e.g. once a month for a couple of months, then make the increments more frequent e.g. every 3 weeks, and then every two weeks.

If you feel able to increment quicker do **but don't over do it!** If you feel you need more time, then do a period without any increments.

Which Cardio

Choose a Cardio you will enjoy doing. If in-doubt, start with walking, as you get fitter move to cycling, as you get even fitter move to Running.

Target (Cardio)

You should aim for 1 to 3 lbs (0.45 to 1.36 kgs) of body fat loss per week. This will be between a 500 calorie and 1500 calorie difference per day. For cardio the target will be 30% of the calorie difference.

Target Fat Loss per week	Cardio changes per day (30%)
0.5 lbs (0.22 kg)	Extra **75** calories of Cardio
1lbs (0.45 kg)	Extra **150** calories of Cardio
1.5 lbs (0.68 kg)	Extra **225** calories of Cardio
2 lbs (0.90 kg)	Extra **300** calories of Cardio
2.5 lbs (1.13 kg)	Extra **375** calories of Cardio
3 lbs (1.36 kg)	Extra **450** calories of Cardio

Calorie Difference Warning

WARNING: Always ensure you consume a minimum of between 1200 and 1800 calories per day. If you consume less than 1200 to 1800 calories over a period of time this will cause your BMR to drop by a large amount and cause you permanent health problems.

Chapter 7: Your Weight-Lifting

Why Weight-Lifting?

Weight-lifting will help in two way. Firstly, it will require calories to perform, so will help you lose fat. Secondly, it will help you build muscle (albeit slowly), which will reduce your body fat percentage and slightly increase the calories your body needs each day (buy very slightly – 5 to 10 calories per day per new pound of muscle added).

Your Weight-Lifting Approach

Your approach to weight-lifting is based on two simple principles:

1. Consistently performing weight-lifting. This will be ensuring you consistently keep moving.

2. Small increments in your weight-lifting. This will ensure over-time you increase the amount of weight you can lift, the number of repetitions you do per a lift, etc.

Your Starting Point

Everybody who reads this book will have their own starting point, whether this is currently no weight-lifting at all, or infrequent weight-lifting, or regular weight-lifting.

Whatever this is, this is your starting point!

Which Weight-Lifting Program

There are endless weight-lifting programs available for free online, (so please search and find one you would like to try). These programs range from full body work-outs three times a week to a different body-part each day.

To get you going there is an example program at the end of this chapter, but please change this to suit youself.

What Are Reps And Sets?

There is a lot of gym terminology, but the most important terms are:

- **Reps:** (short for repetitions), this is just the number of times you perform the movement (e.g. number of times you lift a weight).

- **Sets:** this is a group of 1 or more reps done before a rest break. You may do 8 reps and then rest for 1 minute then do another 8 reps, in this case you have done 2 sets of 8 reps.

- **Working Sets:** performing the movement with your working weight (weight that will strain but not injury you).

- **Warm-up Sets:** performing the movement with a lighter weight to warm-up the muscles. This is very important to prevent injury.

- **Rest Time:** the seconds or minutes you rest between sets. Usually this will be between 30 seconds and 5 minutes.

- **Muscle Group:** collection of muscles (e.g. Back).

- **Split:** how often you train a muscle group, e.g. if you wanted to do 120 reps on your chest. If you worked-out chest 1 time a week you would do 120 reps on that day, and have a '1 day split'. But if you worked-out chest 2 times a week, then you would do 60 reps on each of the two days, and have a '2 day split'.

How Many Reps?

The number of reps per a week, depends on the muscle group, e.g. your back will require more reps than your biceps, because you back muscles are much bigger.

Below is a rough guide (a rule of thumb) to use when you start and then as you learn about your body you can do what is more specific to you.

Muscle Group	Repetitions Per Week	
	Low	High
Chest	60	120
Back	60	120
Quadriceps	60	120
Hamstrings	60	120
Shoulders	30	60
Biceps	30	60
Triceps	30	60
Calves	30	60
Abs	30	60

This is telling you your chest requires between 60 (lower-end) and 120 (higher-end) repetitions per a week.

How Many Sets?

This is where things get a little more tricky, as the number of sets is impacted by the number of times per a week you train that muscle group (your split). But to keep things simple we will assume 10 repetitions per set.

Below is a rough guide (a rule of thumb) to use when you start. As your learn about your body you can do what is more specific to you.

Muscle Group	Sets Per Week	
	Low	High
Chest	6	12
Back	6	12
Quadriceps	6	12
Hamstrings	6	12
Shoulders	3	6
Biceps	3	6
Triceps	3	6
Calves	3	6
Abs	3	6

What Is The Program?

The program for you to start with is as follows:

Day			Exercise	Warm-Up Sets	Working Sets	Weight
				Sets * Reps	Sets * Reps	
			Session 1 – Chest, Shoulders, & Triceps			
Monday & Thursday	1	Chest	Exercise for Chest (e.g. Chest Press)	2 * (6)	3 * (10)	Medium weight with good form
	2	Shoulder	Exercise for Shoulders (e.g. Shoulder Press)	1 * (6)	3 * (10)	
	3	Triceps	Exercise for Triceps (e.g. Tricep Pull-Down)	1 * (6)	3 * (10)	
			Session 3 – Back & Biceps			
Tuesday & Friday	1	Back	Exercise for Back (e.g. Lat Pull-Down)	2 * (6)	3 * (10)	Medium weight with good form
	2	Traps	Exercise for Traps (e.g. Dumbbell Shrugs)	1 * (6)	2 * (10)	
	3	Bicep	Exercise for Biceps (e.g. Bicep Curl)	1 * (6)	3 * (10)	
			Session 1 – Legs			
Wednesday & Saturday	1	Quads	Exercise for Quads (e.g. Squat)	2 * (6)	3 * (10)	Medium weight with good form
	2	Hamstrings	Exercise for Hamstrings (e.g. Lying Leg Curls)	2 * (6)	3 * (10)	
	3	Calves	Exercise for Calves (e.g. Calf Raises)	2 * (6)	3 * (10)	

Interpreting The Program

The program is 6 day a week program. Where you do two Leg days (Wednesday & Saturday); You do two Chest, Shoulder and Triceps days (Monday & Thursday); You do two Back, Traps, and Biceps days (Tuesday & Friday). You can change which days you do which work-out, but ensure you give each muscle group at least 24 hours rest before working-out that same muscle group again.

Lets look at an exercise. For Exercise 1 (for Chest) on Monday & Thursday you will **eventually** be doing:

- Two warm-up sets of the chest exercise. Each warm-up set will be for 6 repetitions.

- Each warm-up set will use a higher weight.

- Three working sets of the chest exercise. Each working set will be for 10 repetitions.

- Rest 30 – 60 seconds between each warm-up and each working sets.

Do I Just Start Everything?

You will start as follows: Doing 2 exercises from each day's work-out, and doing each day's work-out 1 time per week, e.g.:

Phase 1:

- Monday: **You will do 2 exercises**.
- Tuesday: You will do nothing.
- Wednesday: **You will do 2 exercises**.

- Thursday: You will do nothing.
- Friday: **You will do 2 exercises.**
- Saturday: You will do nothing.

Phase 2:

- Monday: **You will do 3 exercises**.
- Tuesday: You will do nothing.
- Wednesday: **You will do 3 exercises**.
- Thursday: You will do nothing.
- Friday: **You will do 3 exercises.**
- Saturday: You will do nothing.

Phase 3:

- Monday: **You will do 3 exercises**.
- Tuesday: **You will do 3 exercises**.
- Wednesday: **You will do 3 exercises**.
- Thursday: **You will do 3 exercises**.
- Friday: **You will do 3 exercises.**
- Saturday: **You will do 3 exercises.**

You can aim to perform Phase 1 for between 1 and 2 months before going to Phase 2. Then aim to perform Phase 2 for between 1 and 2 months before going to Phase 3. Then you will be doing Phase 3 for the rest of the time you are on your journey.

How Often Do I Increment?

Judge this by how you feel doing the phase, but as a rough rule of thumb every 4 to 8 weeks, try to increment to the next phase.

If this is too fast for you, then delay it until you are comfortable. If this is too slow for you, then speed it up.

As you expand you may wish to increase from 3 exercises per work-out to 4 exercises per work-out, and then 5 exercises per work-out.

How Do I Know Which Exercises?

What exercises to do, and videos showing good form are available via searching on-line. This is your next stop. Chapter 12 gives you some recommended web-sites where you can find information on particular exercises.

How Much Weight Do I Use?

Start with a small weight, don't worry how much weight other people are using. When the weight becomes easy then increase the weight.

As a rule of thumb, try to use a weight for your working-set that you can do for 10 reps then you need a rest.

How Often Do I Increase The Weight?

Increase the weight when doing that exercise with that weight for 10 reps becomes easy for you.

How Much Do I Increase The Weight?

When it comes to increasing weight, try to increase the weight by between 5% to 10% at each increment.

Target (Weight-Lifting)

You should aim for 1 to 3 lbs (0.45 to 1.36 kgs) of body fat loss per week. This is between a 500 and 1500 calorie difference per day.

For weight-lifting the target will be 10% of the calorie difference.

Target Fat Loss per week	Weight-lifiting changes per day (10%)
0.5 lbs (0.22 kg)	Extra **25** calories of weight-lifting
1 lbs (0.45 kg)	Extra **50** calories of weight-lifting
1.5 lbs (0.68 kg)	Extra **75** calories of weight-lifting
2 lbs (0.90 kg)	Extra **100** calories of weight-lifting
2.5 lbs (1.13 kg)	Extra **125** calories of weight-lifting
3 lbs (1.36 kg)	Extra **150** calories of weight-lifting

Calorie Difference Warning

WARNING: Always ensure you consume a minimum of between 1200 and 1800 calories per day. If you consume less than 1200 to 1800 calories over a period of time this will cause your BMR to drop by a large amount and cause you permanent health problems.

Chapter 8: Your NEAT

What Is NEAT?

What is NEAT? NEAT standards for **Non-exercise activity thermogenesis** and is all energy expended ([Calories Out]) that is not from sports-like exercise (cardio or weight-lifting) or bodily functions (for example sleeping or eating). This will include things such as dusting, gardening, walking to buy a paper, etc. Think of this as the day-to-day chores you do.

How to measure your NEAT

As NEAT is very complex and therefore very difficult to measure, the simplest approach is to measure the time you perform the following:

- Time spent walking (non-exercise based).
- Time spent performing general tasks, e.g. house work, gardening, etc.

Once you have a rough average daily amount e.g. 35 minutes, you can use this as a basis and build upon this.

Next Step

Measure your NEAT for between 3 and 5 days, recording the amount in time. Then take the average of these measurements.

Your Starting Point

Once you have calculated an average daily amount, this becomes your starting point for NEAT.

Whatever this is, this is your starting point!

How To Increment

Every week you are going to simply increase the amount of time your performing NEAT. This will be as simple as increasing from 35 minutes to 40 minutes of NEAT per day.

Example 1: You currently do 15 minutes of NEAT (dusting), your first 5 increments could be:

- Increment to: 20 minutes of NEAT per day.
- Increment to: 25 minutes of NEAT per day.
- Increment to: 30 minutes of NEAT per day.
- Increment to: 35 minutes of NEAT per day.
- Increment to: 40 minutes of NEAT per day.

Example 2: You currently do 140 minutes of NEAT (gardening, dusting, or shopping) on average per day, your first 5 increments could be:

- Increment to: 145 minutes of NEAT per day.
- Increment to: 150 minutes of NEAT per day.
- Increment to: 155 minutes of NEAT per day.
- Increment to: 160 minutes of NEAT per day.
- Increment to: 165 minutes of NEAT per day.

Increment Types

Do you need to increment a particular type of NEAT? **No!**

You can either increment the amount of your current NEAT activity you are doing, e.g. increase your daily gardening from 15 minutes to 20 minutes. Or you can do an additional NEAT activity, e.g. gardening for 15 minutes plus an additional 5 minutes of walking per day.

Increment Limit

You can increment upto a maximum of 3 additional hours or a total of 6 hours NEAT per day.

Increment Suggestions

Below are some suggestions on ways to increment your NEAT:

1. Start: If you don't currently do a NEAT activity (e.g. gardening) start by doing some.
2. Day-to-day tasks:
   - Increase the time you spend walking around a shop as you do your shopping.
   - Park further away from shops and walk to the shops.
   - Spend more time on house-hold chores.
3. Going to, from and whilst at work:
   - If you get a bus or train, then get-off 1 stop earlier and walk.
   - If you drive, park further away so you walk.

- Always take the stairs rather than the elevator.
- Move more at work, by getting up and speaking to colleagues rather than emailing them.
- Go for a walk at lunch time, or spending your lunch time walking up and down the stairs.

Target (NEAT)

You should aim for 1 to 3 lbs (0.45 to 1.36 kgs) of body fat loss per week. This is between a 500 and 1500 calorie difference per day.

For NEAT the target will be 10% of the calorie difference.

Target Fat Loss per week	NEAT changes per day (10%)
0.5 lbs (0.22 kg)	Extra 25 calories of NEAT
1 lbs (0.45 kg)	Extra 50 calories of NEAT
1.5 lbs (0.68 kg)	Extra 75 calories of NEAT
2 lbs (0.90 kg)	Extra 100 calories of NEAT
2.5 lbs (1.13 kg)	Extra 125 calories of NEAT
3 lbs (1.36 kg)	Extra 150 calories of NEAT

Calorie Difference Warning

WARNING: Always ensure you consume a minimum of between 1200 and 1800 calories per day. If you consume less than 1200 to 1800 calories over a period of time this will cause your BMR to drop by a large amount and cause you permanent health problems.

Chapter 9: Your Sleep

Importance Of Sleep

Sleep is one of the most important aspects to fat loss (or muscle building or body re-composition). It is during sleep that your body does a series of tasks that will aid your journey:

- Uses calories to perform bodily functions for fat loss.

- Builds muscle for increased muscle mass.

- Repairs your body, allowing you to perform cardio and weight-lifting the next day.

Target (Sleep)

You should aim for between 8 hours of sleep and 10 hours of sleep per day. **With 8 hours an absolute minimum.**

Get into a routine of "early" to bed and getting a good nights sleep.

Sleep Tips

Below are so tips to help you get a better nights sleep:

When	Sleep Tip
Before Bed (2-3 hours)	Stop drinking coffee, tea, soda drinks.
Before Bed (1-2 hours)	Stop eating anything.
Before Bed (1-2 hours)	Stop using computer, phone, television.
Before Bed (15-30 minutes)	Goto toilet.
During sleep	Ensure there are no turned on phones or tablets.
During sleep	Ensure your curtains / blinds are pulled to reduce outside light.
During sleep	Dress to ensure you are not too cold or too warm .
Next Morning	Remove duvet or blank and 'air' the bed.
Next Morning	Stretch out for a minute.

Chapter 10: Your Life

Fitting Everything Into Your Life

You have a busy and complicated life, like everyone else who uses this book. Therefore you have to plan to fit all aspects of this approach into your life.

Putting Things Together

Lets break-down your commitment to this approach on a daily basis. It will look a little like the below:

Approach	Daily Time in hours
Meal Preparation	0.5 hours
Cardio	0.5 – 1 hours
Weight-Lifting	0.5 – 1 hours
NEAT	1 – 3 hours
Sleep	8 hours
Commuting (Gym, etc.)	1 – 2 hours

Additionally, your weekly commitment will look like this:

Approach	Daily Time in hours
Shopping	1 – 2 hours
Meal Preparation	1 – 2 hours
Measuring Progress	0.5 hours
Planning next weeks Diet	0.5 hours

So you now need to work-out how to fit all the daily commitments into your busy day:

- 24 hours in a day minus 8 hours for the sleep.
- 16 hours minus work (8hrs) and life commitments (2hrs) leave you with spare time – 6 hours.
- In the spare time (6hrs) you need to fit in between 3 to 6 hours for the Meal Preparation, Cardio, Weight-Lifting, and NEAT.

What To Do If You Do Not Have Enough Time?

The true answer should be: **Make Time!**

But we all live busy lives, so compromise is the best option: **Do some of the approach if you cannot do all of the approach!**

If you cannot commit to doing all activities for the correct amount of time, try some of the below, starting at the top and only doing the last two points if you **absolutely** have to:

1. **Make extra time:** Reduce or remove time spent watching TV, on the internet, hobbies, etc. to make extra time. **You health is more important than a TV program!**
2. Reduce your calorie difference and extend the time: This will mean you need to do less per day.
3. **Use your work:** Try to combine your cardio, NEAT, and weight-lifting with your work, for example:
   - Could you walk or cycle to work or walk or cycle during your lunch time (cardio)?
   - Is there a gym close to work for a lunch-time work-out (weight-lifting)?

- Can you do more NEAT as part of work?
- Can you put a mini-exercise bike or mini-stepper under your desk and use it while you work?

4. **Use Time Better:** For example could you:
   - Walk or cycle to the gym for cardio? So you use the gym for just weight-lifting.
   - Walk or cycle to shops, etc. as cardio?

5. **Substitute:** Can you save time (e.g. commuting to the gym) by substituting gym exercises for home exercises (you will have to buy some dumbbells for use at home)?

6. **Reduced Activity Time:** Do all activities for less time, e.g. rather than 1 hours cardio, do 0.5 hours cardio; rather than 3 hours NEAT do 2 hours NEAT.

7. **Drop Activities:** If you **ABSOLUTELY** have to, drop activities in this order:
   1. Weight-Lifting is the first to drop.
   2. NEAT is the second to drop.
   3. Cardio should be the last item to drop.

Whatever you situation, you **cannot** and **must not** cut down or drop the following:

- Diet. *This includes shopping and meal preparation.*
- Sleep. *Minimum 8 hours a day.*

Can You Just Do One Part Of The Approach?

Can you just do one part of the approach, e.g. just do a diet or just do cardio? This is possible, but not recommended as if you fail at that one activity, then you fail full-stop!

If you must take this approach, then focus on Diet first, and when you get time (even the odd hour at weekends) then do cardio & weight-lifting

Chapter 11: Your Progress

Measuring Your Progress

It is important you measure your progress. This will show you that you are making progress and heading towards your target.

Seeing progress increases motivation, which in-turn increases your determination to get to your target.

How To Measure Your Progress

How you measure your progress, will depend on your current point, and where you want to get to. Some ideas are:

1. Recording your weight in pounds (lbs).

2. Recording your waist circumference (around the belly-button) in centimeters (cm).

3. Recording your Hip circumference (widest point) in centimeters (cm).

4. Photos, showing front, side, and back pictures of your body. *Depending on where you are and how comfortable you are doing this.*

How Often To Measure Your Progress

Keep this simple. Record your measurements **one time per week**. This way it is regular enough to see progression, but not too often to become a chore.

How To Record Progression

A simple spreadsheet recording the date, weight, waist measurement, hip measurement, and a goal:

Date	Weight (lbs.)	Waist (cm.)	Hip (cm.)	Goals	Met Goal
12/07/2019	205 lbs	112 cm	134 cm	Weigh less than or equal to 203 lbs	No.
19/07/2019	204 lbs	112 cm	133 cm	Weigh less than or equal to 203 lbs	Yes.
26/07/2019	203 lbs	112 cm	133 cm	No chocolate next week.	Yes.
02/08/2019	201 lbs	111 cm	132 cm	Increase Squat by 10%	Yes.
09/08/2019					
16/08/2019					
23/08/2019					
30/08/2019					
06/09/2019					

Why Include A Goal?

Setting a weekly goal will give you something to aim for next week. This will help to motivate and focus you. The goal can be against a series of factors:

- Your measurements: to weight a certain amount, or for your waist or hips to measure a certain amount.

- Your diet: for example, 'do not eat any chocolate this week'.

- Your cardio: for example, 'complete 5 x 25 minute cycling sessions this week'.

- Your weight-lifting: for example, 'increase chest exercise by 1 repetition'.

- Your NEAT activity: for example, 'get-off 1 bus stop early and walk to my location'.

How Many Goals

How many goals can you set each week?

A maximum of one goal per week!

You need to keep things simple, and not push yourself too hard. So each week you can set upto one goal per week. Setting more than one goal will just cause you to focus on too much at once.

Chapter 12: Tips

Tips To Help You On Your Journey

Below are some tips and tricks to help you on your journey. Do not try to implement every tip & trick from day 1, rather introduce each tip & trick over time, as and when you need them.

Some tips & tricks you will find more helpful and more practical for you, than other tips & tricks.

No.	Tip	Why?
1	Drink 1 pint of water (0.5 litres) or water as soon as you wake up	This will feel you up, so you are not hungry when you go down to the kitchen.
2	Drink 1 pint of water (0.5 litres) or water 15 minutes before each meal.	This will feel you up, so you eat less.
3	Eat on smaller plates.	Small plates will make the meal appear bigger.
4	Chew each mouthful 15 times.	This slows down your consumption time, and will make you feel fuller.
5	Swap White bread for Wholegrain bread.	This will have more fibre to keep you fuller.
6	Add low calorie fillers to meals (Breakfasts): - Blueberries, raspberries, or strawberries to cereals.	This will give you more food for not too many more calories.
7	Add low calorie fillers to meals (Lunches): - Lettuce, Carrots, Celery, Cucumber, or Tomatoes in sandwiches.	This will give you more food for not too many more calories.
8	Add low calorie fillers to meals (Dinners): - Baked Potatoes with main-meals.	This will give you more food for not too many more calories.
9	Keep high-calorie food (Chocolate; Crisps; Biscuits; Cakes; etc.) out-of-sight.	To avoid temptation.
10	When buying food, buy what you need, do not buy extra because it is on offer/better value.	This will avoid over eating.
11	Eat regular smaller meals.	So you are constantly re-fuelling
12	When you crave 'sweet' things eat fruit (Apples; Oranges; Bananas; Strawberries; Raspberries; etc.)	These are lower calorie than chocolate/sweets/biscuits/etc.
13	Have healthy snacks available all the time: Celery, Carrot sticks, Cucumber sticks, Apple pieces.	In-case you need food.
14	Don't have food on your desk at work. Put it out-of-sight.	This will prevent constant snacking.
15	If you miss one cardio session make sure you do it the next time.	This will stop you crashing off the process.
16	If you miss one weight-lifting session make sure you do it the next time.	This will stop you crashing off the process.
17	If you mess-up your diet, make sure you stick to the diet the next day.	This will stop you crashing off the process.

100 Calorie Snacks

Below are some snacks which are roughly 100 calories. You can use these as snacks, or when you desperately need something to eat.

Also, you can take 3 or 4 '100 calorie snack' items to make-up a 300 – 400 calorie meal.

Meal	Current	Estimated Calories
Snack	25g of porridge & water.	100
Snack	40g Yoghurt	100
Snack	Banana (Medium)	100
Snack	Apple	75
Snack	Orange	60
Snack	3 Rice Cakes (plain)	90
Snack	2 Rice Cakes (Chocolate)	80
Snack	1 Rice Cakes (plain) and 15g of Peanut Butter	100
Snack	Carrot (200g)	85
Snack	Celery (1000g)	100
Snack	Lettuce (1000g)	100
Snack	Potatoes (90g)	100
Snack	Broccoli (250g)	100
Snack	Brazil Nuts (12g)	100
Snack	Almonds (12g)	100
Snack	2 Boiled Eggs	100
Snack	200g of Fresh Soup	100
Snack	Sugar Free Low Calorie Jelly (25g)	25 – 100
Snack	1 Piece of Toast	100
Snack	Half a Bagel	100

200 Calorie Snacks

Below are some snacks which are roughly 200 calories. You can use these as snacks, and again you can take 2 or 3 '200 calorie snack' items to make-up a 400 – 600 calorie meal.

Meal	Current	Estimated Calories
Snack	50g of porridge & water.	200
Snack	Banana (Large)	150
Snack	Apple (2)	150
Snack	Orange (3)	180
Snack	6 Rice Cakes (plain)	180
Snack	5 Rice Cakes (Chocolate)	200
Snack	3 Rice Cakes (plain) and 20g of Peanut Butter	200
Snack	Carrot (400g)	170
Snack	Celery (2000g)	200
Snack	Lettuce (2000g)	200
Snack	Potatoes (180g)	200
Snack	Broccoli (500g)	200
Snack	Brazil Nuts (25g)	200
Snack	Almonds (25g)	200
Snack	4 Boiled Eggs	200
Snack	400g of Fresh Soup	200
Snack	2 Sugar Free Low Calorie Jelly (25g)	50 – 200
Snack	2 Piece of Toast	200
Snack	1 Bagel	150

100 Calorie Workouts

Below are some work-outs which are roughly 100 calories for a person weighing 150 lbs. Also calories are given for a 200 lbs, a 250 lbs, and a 300 lbs person.

If you weigh more increase the calories (1 calorie per 2 lbs of weight), if you weigh less reduce the calories (1 calorie per 2 lbs of weight).

These are rough estimate of calories burned and are to give you a rough guide.

Exercise	Time-span (minutes)	Estimated Calories used			
		150 lb person	200 lb person	250 lb person	300 lb person
Weight lifting	25 – 35	100	125	150	175
Cycling (stationary bike)	20	100	125	150	175
Dancing	20 – 25	100	125	150	175
Tai Chi	20	100	125	150	175
Walking (slow pace)	30 – 35	100	125	150	175
Walking (medium pace)	20 -25	100	125	150	175
Walking (fast pace)	15 – 20	100	125	150	175
Tennis	15	100	125	150	175
Running (medium pace)	15 – 20	100	125	150	175
Running (fast pace)	10 – 15	100	125	150	175
Sprinting	5 – 10	100	125	150	175
Walking Up and Down Stairs	15 – 20	100	125	150	175
Swimming	10 – 15	100	125	150	175
Gardening	25 – 30	100	125	150	175
Mowing Lawn	20 – 25	100	125	150	175
Rowing	10 – 15	100	125	150	175
Sleeping	180 – 300	100	125	150	175

Helpful Websites

Below are some helpful websites. These websites will be of use to you through-out your journey, so don't rush to absorb all the information they have immediately on day 1, rather use them as 'goto' sources when you need them:

Category	Website	Comment
Nutrition	http://www.myfitnesspal.com/	Good
Nutrition	http://scoobysworkshop.com/	Good
Nutrition	https://evilcyber.com/	Ok
Cardio	http://scoobysworkshop.com/	Good
Cardio	https://evilcyber.com/	Ok
Weight-lifting	https://www.bodybuilding.com/exercises/	Good
Weight-lifting	http://scoobysworkshop.com/	Ok
Weight-lifting	https://evilcyber.com/	Ok
Tools	https://www.myfitnesspal.com/tools/bmr-calculator	Ok

Further Information

What is a Calorie?

A Calorie (or Cal) is defined as a unit of measurement for the energy needed to raise the temperature of an amount of water. There are in-fact two types of Calories **Small Calories** and **Large (or Food) Calories**. Each type of Calorie raises a different amount of water by 1°C, Small Calories raise 1 gram of water by 1°C; Large (or Food) Calories raise 1 kg (1000 grams) of water by 1°C.

What is a Kilocalorie?

A Kilocalorie (or Kcal) is again a unit of measurement for the energy needed to raise the temperature of an amount of water. The relationship between Kilocalories and Calories is 1 Kcal is equal to 1000 small Cals; 1 Kcal is equal to 1 Large (or Food) Calorie.

BMR or RMR

BMR - Basal Metabolic Rate

RMR – Resting Metabolic Rate

The amount of calories that your body needs just to keep you alive is known as the Basal Metabolic Rate (BMR) or the Resting Metabolic Rate (RMR). Of the two RMR is consider the most accurate.

Calories Percentage Breakdown

As a general overview (not specific to anyone and give as a guide), the breakdown of the percentage of calories consumed is as follows:

| Task | Comment | Estimated Percentage | |
		Low activity person	High activity person
BMR	All tasks to keep your body functioning at rest.	85%	55%
TEF	Thermic effect of food (energy to consume food)	10%	10%
NEAT	Non-Exercise activity thermogenesis e.g. day-to-day activities like gardening.	5%	20%
EAT	Exercise activity thermogenesis e.g. going for a run or walking	0%	15%

As you can see Exercising will only consume a small amount of the calories (ranging from 0 to 15%), this I why the recommend approaches to fat loss in this book work on **nutrition and exercise**.

Calories Per Macronutrients

Below is a break-down of the number of calories in 1g of the macronutrients. As you can see Fat and Alcohol are the most calorie dense (number of calories per a gram).

Macronutrient	Calories Per
Fat	9
Ethanol (alcohol)	7
Carbohydrates	4
Protein	4

Calories Per Food Component

Below is a break-down of the number of calories in 1g of the various food components. As you can see Fat and Alcohol are the most calorie dense (number of calories per a gram).

Food Component	Calories per gram
Fat	9
Ethanol (alcohol)	7
Carbohydrates	4
Protein	4
Organic Acids	3
Polyols (Sugar alcohol)	2.4
Fiber	2

Micronutrients

Below is a break-down of the micronutrients.

Micronutrient
Boron
Cobalt
Chromium
Copper
Fluoride
Iodine
Iron
Manganese
Molybdenum
Selenium
Zinc

RDA or GDA

RDA – Recommended Daily Allowance.

GDA – Guideline Daily Allowance.

Recommended Daily Allowance (RDA) and Guideline Daily Allowance (GDA) are the recommendations on how many calories an individual should consume each day, and are the same thing. The basic recommendations are:

Person	RDA / GDA
Child (Female & Male)	1500
Adult (Female)	2000
Adult (Male)	2500

Why RDAs Are Flawed

Recommended Daily Allowance (and GDA) values are flawed for the reason that they are not unique to individuals. As an example, lets' look at two people:

- **Person A** is an 18 year old Male who exercises for 2 hours a day, walks 1.5 hours a day, is a construction worker and is 195 lbs. According to the RDA Person A needs 2500 Calories a day.

- **Person B** is a 45 year old Male who does no physical activity, is a bus driver and is 140 lbs. According to the RDA Person B needs 2500 Calories a day.

You should see that the RDA has a problem. How can two people, with vastly differing ages; weight; activity levels; etc. need the exact same number of calories?

TDEE

TDEE – Total Daily Energy Expenditure

The TDEE stands for Total Daily Energy Expenditure and is all the calories used by you that day - Calories out. Covering everything from Brain to Bodily Functions to Activities to Exercise. Your TDEE is specific to you and specific to that day, e.g. on Monday you might have a TDEE of 2750 Calories and on Wednesday need 3000 Calories (as you did more exercise) and on Sunday only need 2200 Calories as you did less. Remember this is the Total **Daily** Energy Expenditure e.g. Calories Out for that day.

Aerobic Exercises

Aerobic exercises include cycling, walking, running, hiking, playing football, playing tennis, sprinting, etc. and focus on cardiovascular workouts.

Anaerobic Exercises

Anaerobic exercises include weight lifting, strength training, and resistance training.

Reduce The Calories In (Consumed)

This will involve reducing the amount and kinds of food and drink you consume to ensure the total number of calories you consume each day is less than your body requires so you loss fat.

This is the fastest way to lose fat.

Increase The Calories Out (Expended)

This is achieved by being more active, meaning starting or increasing your Aerobic exercises (cardio – walking, cycling, running, playing tennis, etc.), which is the most effective way. You can see similar result, but much less, via Anaerobic exercises (weight-lifting). This is achieved by increasing your TDEE.

Increase BMR

You can increase your BMR by increasing your muscle mass.

This is a very slow way to lose fat. Muscle takes months and years to build and the increase in BMR is very small. As an example 1 pound of muscle will take at least 1 month to build and 1 pound of muscle will increase your BMR by around 8 calories a day.

Thermodynamics.

Your body needs to be kept at a consistent temperature from 97°F (36.1°C) to 99°F (37.2°C), with the average temperature being 98.6°F (37°C). If your body has lower temperature your body has to work harder to warm you up; if your body has a higher temperature your body has to work harder to cool you down. If you ran 1 mile in winter in cold-climate running gear you will burn less calories than if you ran the same distance naked.

You can use temperature changes to help your fat loss, but it risks health issues and is **NOT** advised.

This is a very slow way to lose fat and risks hurting your health. Please do not do this.

Support

Feedback And Help

Please feel free to provide feedback on this book or ask questions, by emailing **simpleapproachto@gmail.com** and I will try to help you as best I can.

Other Services

If you would like to purchase a tailor-made diet program, meal options, or training program, then please email **simpleapproachto@gmail.com** and I will provide you with a list of options.

www.ingramcontent.com/pod-product-compliance
Lightning Source LLC
Chambersburg PA
CBHW021240280526
45784CB00005B/2171